*Autograph*

*Heart problems*

*every one should know*

Copyright © 2024 by Hashmat Rajput. "Heart problems every one should know."

All rights reserved. This book is fully protected by US copyright laws. No form of this book is reproduced by copying, photocopying, scanning, digital or any other modern means. Certificate of Registration is TXu2-445-989.
ISBN:

Printed in the United States of America.

# HEART

## PROBLEMS EVERY ONE SHOULD KNOW

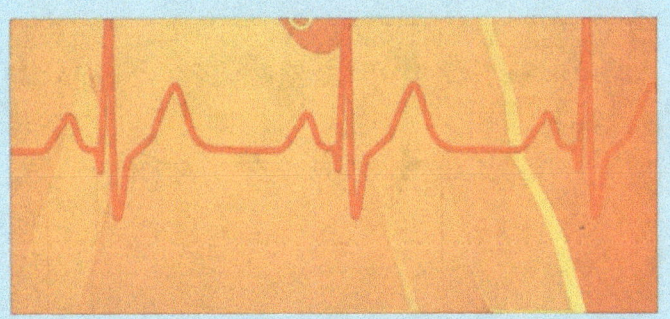

**H. A. RAJPUT, MD. FACP.**

# Acknowledgment

I would like to acknowledge my sincere thanks to CANVA and it's team with contributors, and supporters who provided the graphics and photos for this book.

This book is dedicated to my parents,
my wife, and my children.
Of course, to my patients,
who are always my family.

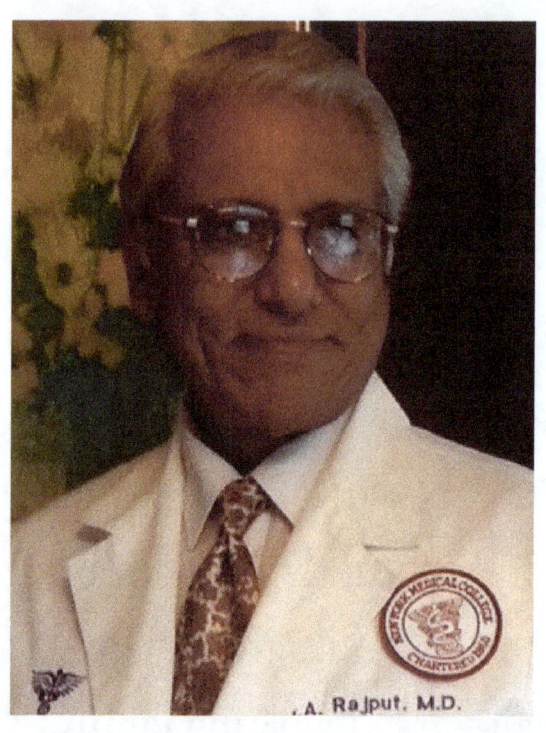

**Hashmat A. Rajput, MD. FACP.**

amazon.com/author/doctorrajput
bit.ly/3YK1Vxf
hashmatrajput@facebook.cm
x.comdr4urhealth
www.pinterest.com/hashmat rajput
hshmatrajput@threads.net
https://www.youtube.com/@hashmatrajput1123
drhashmatrajput@linkedin.com

I am Dr. Rajput from New York and have the great pleasure of introducing myself to you. I'm passionate about Internal Medicine and have a great experience in the prevention, diagnosis, and treatment of diseases. My experience involves working in the hospitals, nursing homes, private offices, and even house calls. Health Tap is a national Telehealth company in the United States of America, and I earned the title of Thought Leader of New York by my contributions.

Currently I am a Senior Attending Physician at Phelps Memorial Hospital Center of Northwell Health, and Assistant Professor of Clinical Medicine at New York Medical College. I am A proud Fellow member of the American College of Physicians, USA.

I made tremendous differences in the lives of my patients. I love to help each human being medically, who comes in contact with me. This is my life mission, and I wish you the best of health.

# CONTENTS
## CHEST PAIN-12

1. HEART ATTACK-16
2. ANGINA-29
3. AORTIC ANEURYSM-33
4. PERICARDITIS-38
5. PULMONARY EMBOLISM-52

# CONTENTS

6. PNEUMONIA-62

7. PNEUMOTHORAX-66

8. PEPTIC ULCER-70

9. ACID REFLUX-77

10. GALLSTONE-84

11. COSTOCHONDRITIS-91

12. ANXIETY-96

# HEART

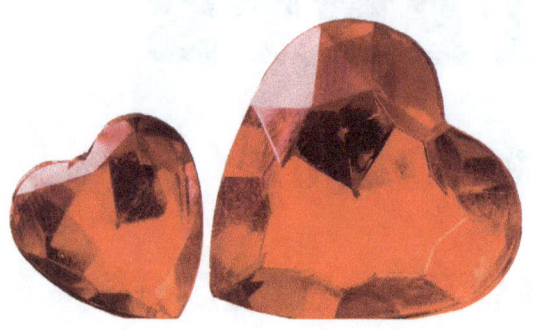

It is a vital organ for the life. It is a muscular pump in our body which circulates the pure oxygenated blood via arteries and capillaries to the cell level. The deoxygenated blood is brought back by veins.

# The oxygen is life.

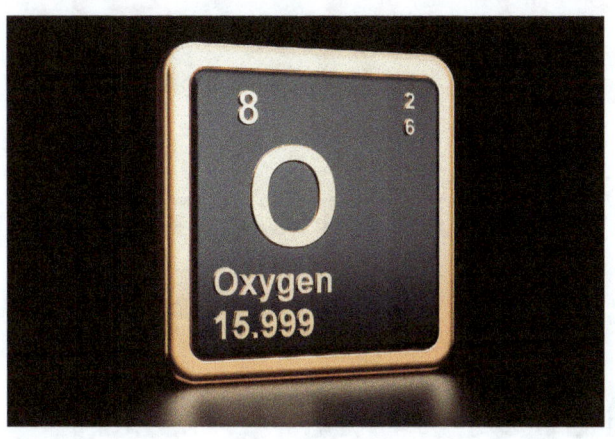

It goes in by breathing into lungs where it combines with red blood cells, and the heart pumps it to the cellular level. The cell breaks the food into energy which is required to survive. with out 4 minutes of oxygen, the death is eminent.

# CHEST PAIN

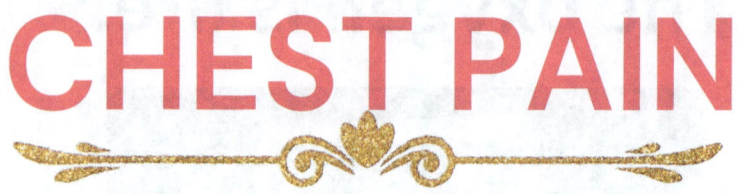

Chest pain can happen at any time, and any where. It can be present in the breast bone, shoulder, arm, or back. The intensity can be mild, moderate, or severe. It can radiate from one part of the body to the other.

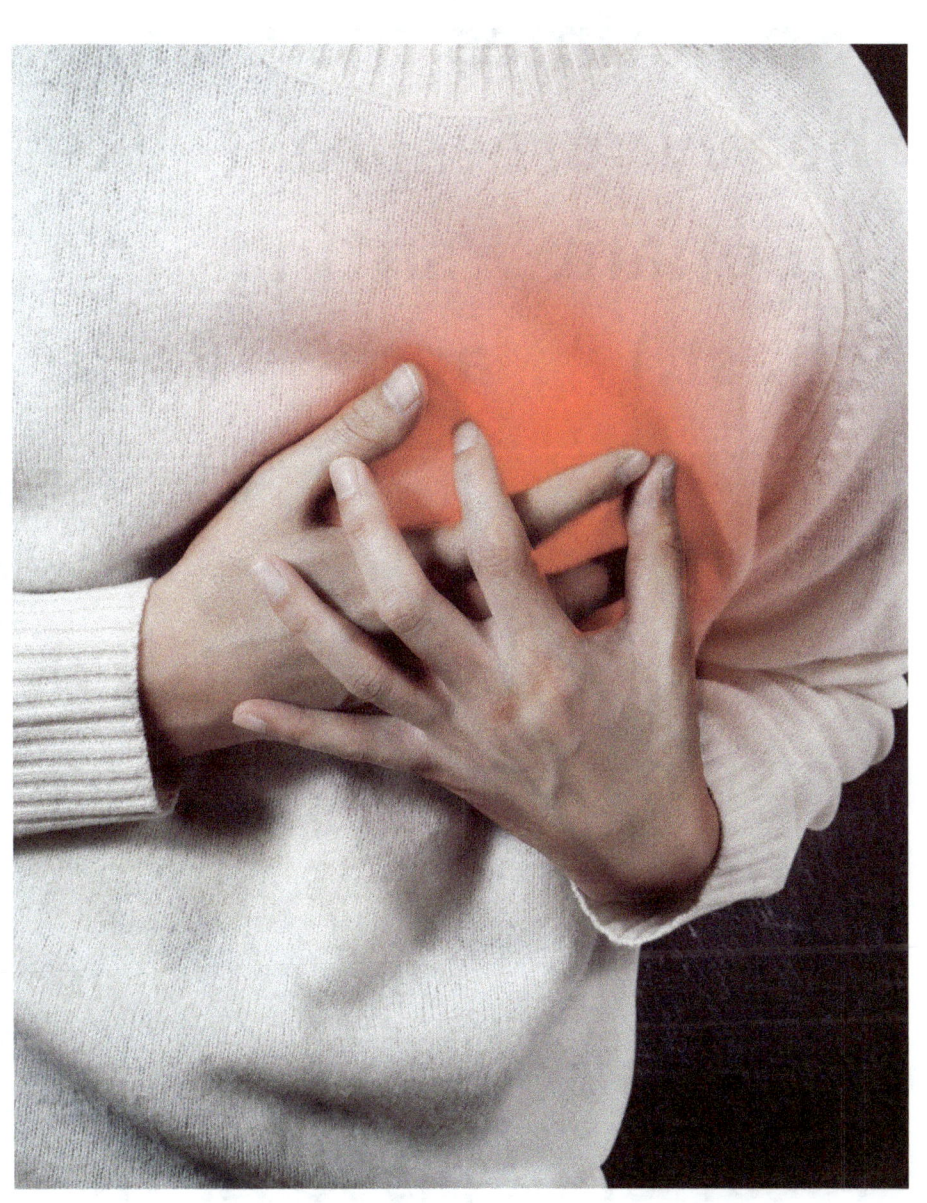

**CHEST PAIN**

13

Sometimes the pain is heavy pressure ( like elephant sitting on chest.) and knife cutting.

It may be associated with nausea, vomitting and passing out. It can be acute or chronic with episodes. It can be recurrent episodes. The patient may collapse or die.

Causes of chest pain:

**HEART ATTACK:**

It is also known as MI (MYOCARDIAL INFARCTION). It is caused by blockage of arteries due to build up of cholesterol plaque and rupture. The plaque is formed by eating fatty foods. The arteries supply blood oxygen to heart itself.

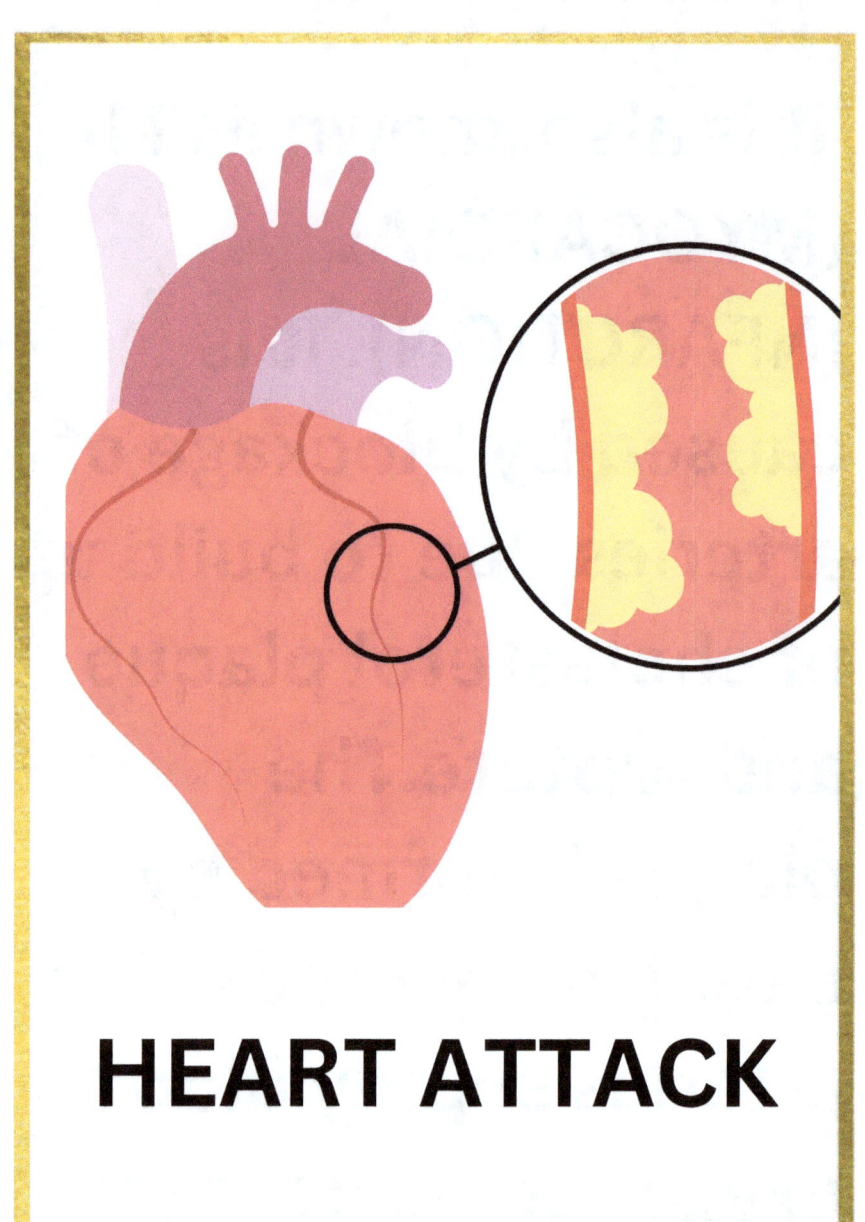

**HEART ATTACK**

If OXYGEN blood supply stops, then that portion of heart tissue becomes ischemic and dies. Oxygen comes from air we breathe in and mixes with red blood cells in the lungs. From lungs it goes into the heart which pumps it through out body at the tissue cellular level. The cell creates energy for life.

The pain is acute or severe. Present in chest, jaw, shoulder, left arm, both arms, or stomach area. it lasts more than 30 minutes. It can be associated with nausea, vomiting, sweating, anxiety, fast heart beats, weakness, tiredness and dizziness. Women present with other symptoms more than chest pain.

The other contributing factors are:
- Unhealthy sedentary life
- Obesity
- Smoking
- Alcohol use
- Drug use
- Blood pressure
- Age
- Diabetes

The process involves the fat deposit in blood vessel with plaque formation. The plaque has a fibrous cap which ruptures and the clot is formed. This clot grows in size and blocks blood supply to heart tissue, causing necrosis. It can be spasm due to cocaine drug use, trauma or vasculitis.

The diagnosis is made with vitals, history and physical examination. Vital signs are blood pressure, pulse rate, respiration rate, temperature, pulse oximeter oxygen, weight. History will be for nature, location, duration of pain and associated symptoms. Exam of heart.

Diagnostic tests: Complete blood count(CBC), comprehensive metabolic panel(CMP), CK-MBI, Troponin, Myoglobin, LDH. Arterial blood gas. ECG to confirm and differentiate Between ST elevation MI (STEMI) vs Non ST elevated MI (NSTEMI) and heart rhythm.

Chest X-ray shows size and fluid, if any. 2DEcho of heart may show , heart and valvular function, size and disease. MRI shows damaged ischemic heart tissues.
Right heart cath. to measure heart and lung pressures.

Angioplasty, instead of clot buster, for blood flow and pain relief.

**Treatment:**
Initially managed by the paramedics in the field, or in the Emergency room by physician, or in the hospital. If the patient is with low blood pressure, irregular heart beat, or nconsciousness, the Cardiopulmonary resuscitation (CPR) is done at home, in transit by paramedics, or in ER.

The basic principle is to maintain ABC airway, breathing and circulation . For protection of airway, the patient is intubated and oxygen is supplied. OXYGEN is constantly monitored. Intravenous lines are placed in, to give initial heart medications. Every one should learn CPR.

In hospital the patient receives blood thinner like Aspirin, Plavix or Heparin. Clot busters like Streptokinase, Alteplase/Tenecteplase and etc. It is given 3-6 hours for optimal results. It can be given up to 12 hours after the onset of chest pain. Continuous oxygen therapy is given.

- Pain management. Aspirin for pain as it prevents further blood clot formation. Do not use Tylenol, Naprosyn or Advil. Morphine is used in severe pain.

Blood thinners. Nitroglycerine to dilate the blood vessels. Also, relieves the chest pain. The cholestrol drugs like Lipitor/Zocor are given.

PLAN:
1. Call 911 ( IN USA).
2. Relax, rest, sit down.
3. Tell some one nearby, your condition.
4. Take one ASPIRIN
5. In case of rural area, ask some one to drive you to ER.

Time is of the essence. The sooner you reach the hospital, the better chances of survival.

# ANGINA:

It is a chronic serious condition. The pain intensity is variable with episodes, and lasts less than 30 minutes. The Cholestrol plaque formation causes the narrowing of the arteries with less blood oxygen supply. Some times it is spasm.

The pain is precipitated with stress, cold, anxiety and heavy work. It is relieved with rest, Nitroglycerine (NTG) and Calcium channel blocker medication. The cause is coronary artery disease with narrowing and less oxygen supply. The heart does not get enough oxygen to work.

Diagnosis of angina is made with signs and symptoms, history physical examination. Also your doctor may give you NTG to see if your pain is relieved. do blood test, STRESS Tread mill test or Nuclear stress test, ECG, 2D ECHO of heart, CT SCAN, MRI and CORONARY ANGIO if needed.

Take the rest and also, NTG as prescribed. If pain does not go away in 5 minutes, take and other dose and go to the hospital. Also, see the primary doctor for medication adjustment and the diagnostic tests. These are Stress test, ECG, AND 2 DECHO of the heart. Change life style. Avoid stress & anxiety.

## AORTIC ANEURYSM:

Aorta is the largest blood tube (vessel) that runs from the left side of heart and carries the oxygenated blood to all parts of the body. It makes an arch coming out of the heart with proximal and distal ends. The distal end becomes the abdominal aorta. The wall of aorta become thin and baloon like, and ruptures very easily.

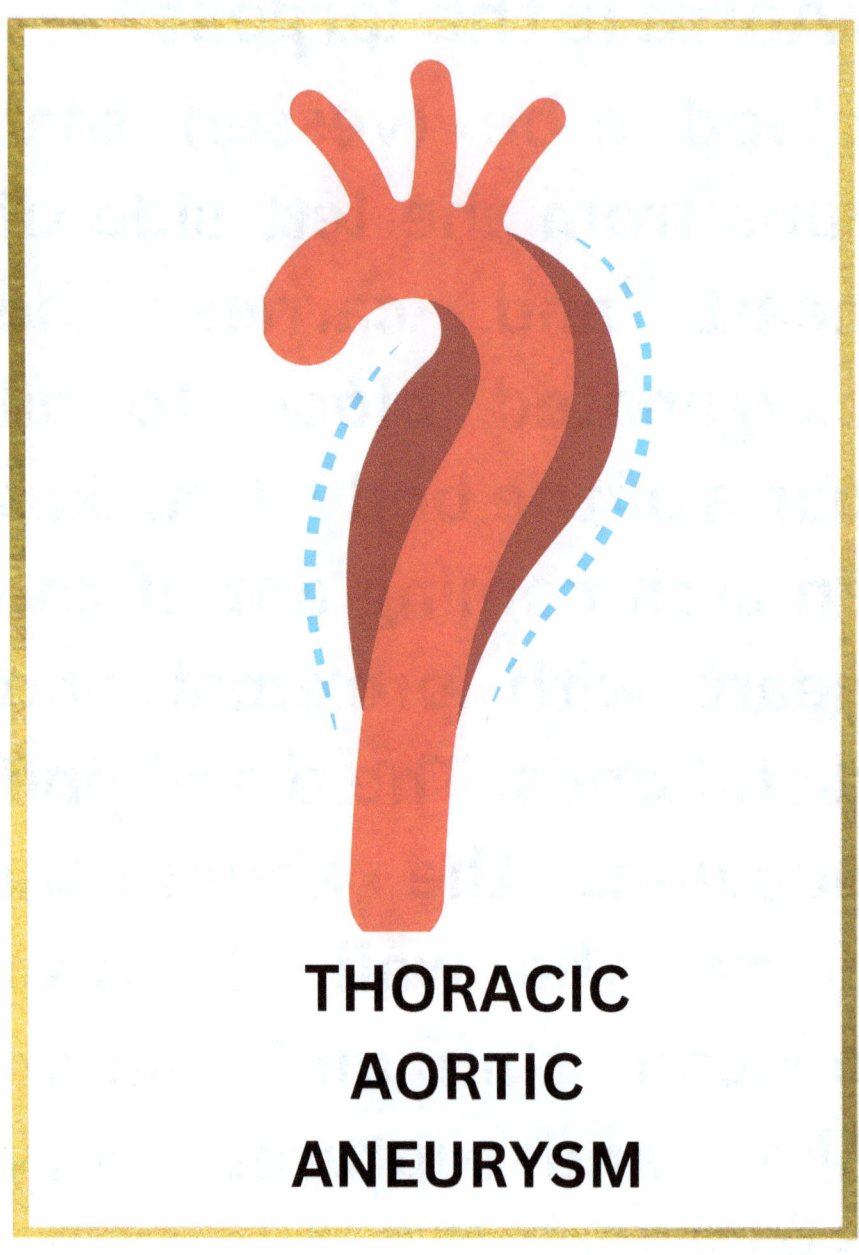

**THORACIC AORTIC ANEURYSM**

Initially asymptomatic.
It is incidental finding on chest x-ray.
CT with contrast for accurate size measurement, is done.
The person may have cough, hoarseness, dyspnea, front and back pain.
Hypotension with shock when it ruptures.

The causes of thoracic aortic aneurysm are:
- Atherosclerosis
- Connective tissue diseases
- Marfan's syndrome
- Hypertension
- Trauma
- Bicuspid valve
- Pregnancy
- Syphilis

When it ruptures, the pain is sudden, excruciating, stabbing, tearing- like knife cutting, in the back. initially the person has different pulse pressure. Later on, progresses to shock with the neurological deficits

**IT IS A TRUE MERGENCY. RUSH TO THE ER. HAS LOW SURVIVAL RATE.**

# PERICARDITIS

The fibrous sac around the heart is called pericardium. It maintains the shape and function of heart. It consists of two layers and the fluid, is in between them. It is supplied with the phrenic nerve. The inflammation of pericardium is called the pericarditis.

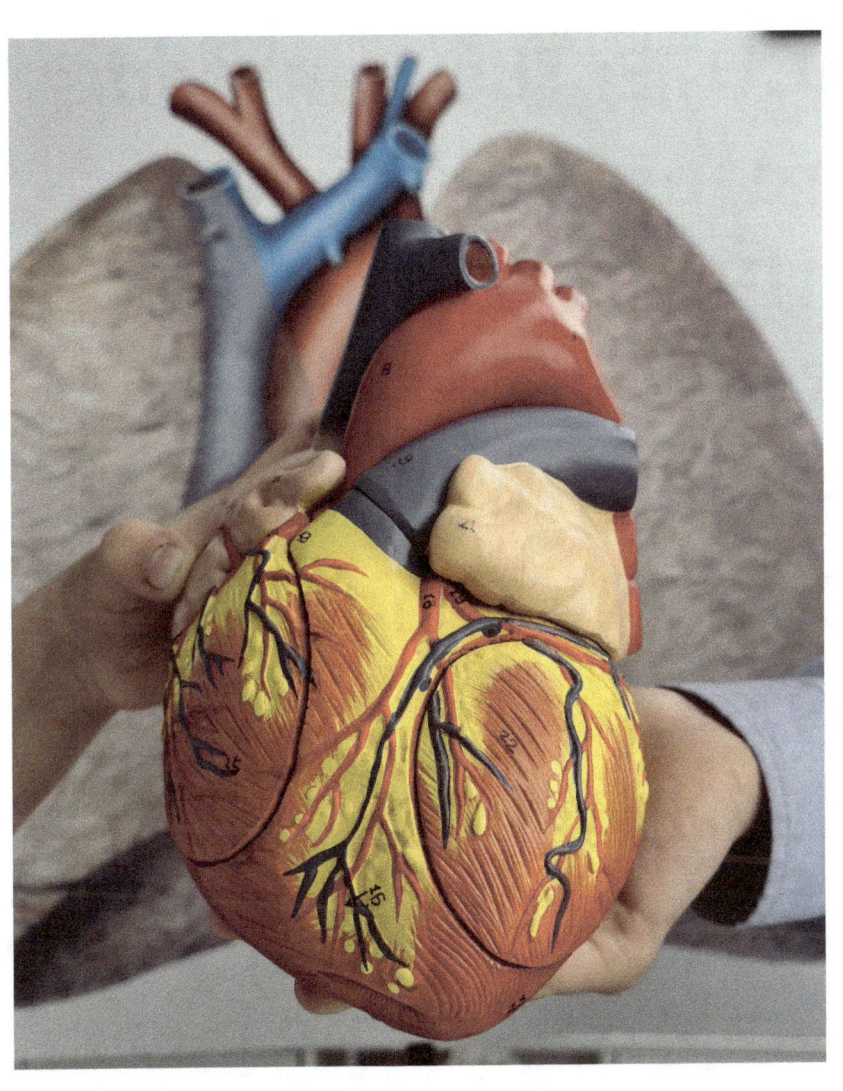

# PERICARDITIS

39

It can be:
ACUTE: The symptoms are less than 6 week.
SUBACUTE: The symptoms are between 6 weeks to 3 months.
CHRONIC: The symptoms are more than 3 months.
RECURRENT: The symptoms come back after initial episode resolution.

Signs and symptoms of Pericarditis include severe sharp stabbing pain in chest ,radiating to left shoulder or arm. The pain gets worse in lying or coughing. It is relieved with sitting and leaning forward. Also may have hoarseness, leg edema, and fast heart beat.

May have fever, weakness, shortness of breath or dizziness. The causes of pericarditis are: INFECTION. It can be viral, bacterial, fungus or parasite. T.B. is the common cause of pericarditis world wide. CANCERS of the lung, colon, melanoma, lymphoma, prostate, etc. can cause it as well.

RADIATION therapy may cause even constrictive pericarditis

INFLAMMATORY DISEASE . Rheumatoid arthritis, Lupus, Scleroderma or Rheumatic fever.

CHEST INJURY car accident.

After MI or heart bypass surgery, valve surgery or pace maker insertion.

**Metabolic diseases:**
Kidney failure
Hypothyroidism
Hypercholestrolemia

**Drugs:**
Phenytoin
Procainamide
Hydralazine, etc.

**Idiopathic:**
The cause is unknown

Diagnosis is made by history and physical examination with pain nature, location and duration.

Presence of friction rub sound on stethoscope. CBC and rheumatic factor for anemia & rheumatic disease. ECG shows ST elevation or PR depression.

Diagnosis of pericarditis requires two of the three elements from chest pain, friction rub and ECG changes. ESR- (erythrocyte sedimentation rate) for inflammation.

CRP( C reactive protein) for inflammation.

CHEST X-ray may show large heart and fluids in the lungs.

MRI-(magnetic resonance imaging) with gadolinium contrast for enhancement of sharp image. 2-DECHO of heart to evaluate heart and valvular function with EJECTION FRACTION. PERICARDIOCENTESIS. It is putting needle in heart and drain fluid.

The fluid drawn, releases the pressure on heart, and also sent for diagnostic sampling.

Initial treatment of pericarditis is Ibuprofen (Motrin or Advil) for 2 weeks. If the symptoms do not resolve, then switch to Colchicine(Colcrys or Mitigare).

If the person is allergic to above medications, then give Prednisone (Deltasone) with care and monitoring.
Treat the above mentioned underlying diseases.
Discontinue the offending drugs. Antibiotics Vancomycin and Ceftriaxone are given for suspected bacterial infection.

# Cradiac TAMPONADE

is the condition of fluid and blood accumulation in pericardium. The heart is comPressed and can not function. This is real emergency and quick pericardiocentesis is done. The needle is inserted and fluid taken out.

*Chest window* is made if tube is not working.

- *Pericardiectomy* is the surgical procedure for removing the sac which is stiff, in *CONSTRICTIVE PERICARDITIS*. The heart can not expand in stiff sac. people recover 2 weeks to 3 months after surgery.

# PULMONARY EMBOLISM

This is a clot in the artery of the lung, blocking the supply of blood and oxygen. It causes sudden death. It originates in the leg veins, and travels from there to the lungs. It is called deep vein thrombosis or (DVT), that happens suddenly in one leg. The veins are iliac, femoral, and popliteal. There is sudden swelling of one calf leg.

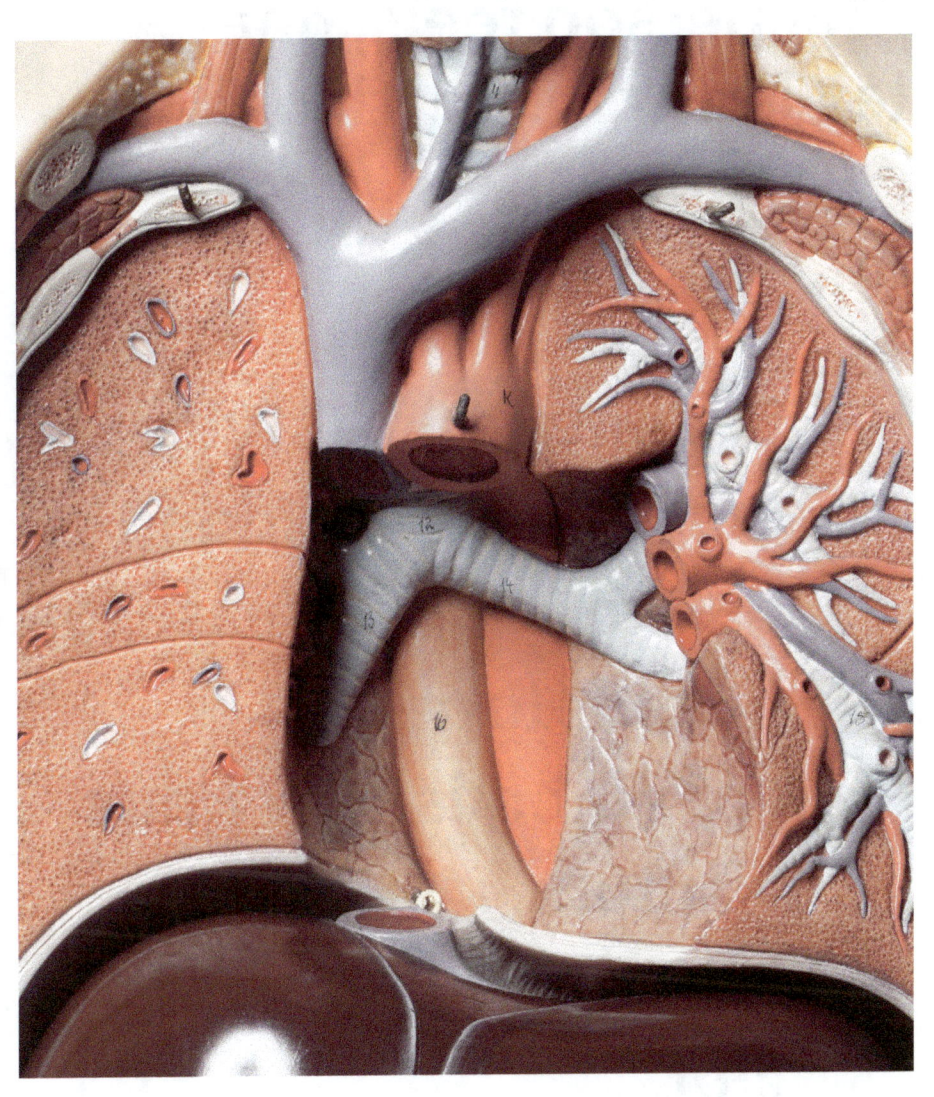

# PULMONARY EMBOLISM

The person feels, one leg is swollen with or without pain.
The causes are:

- Sedentary life style, inactivity, bedridden due to some disease, or hospitalization.
- Fat embolism by bone fracture.
- Iv catheter induced clot.
- Air embolism by surgery, or ventilation.

Any one sitting in car, plane or train more than four hours, is prone to clot formation. One baby aspirin should be taken before trip.

Other causes are: Obesity, with venous stasis.

Post MI, due to weak heart.
CHF, with slow blood flow.
Old age with multiple factors
Trauma, bone fracture.
Cancer and chemotherapy.
Pregnancy, birth control pill
Surgery of abdomen & pelvis
Family history of clot.

The sign and symptoms are unilateral large calf swelling and tenderness on dorsiflexion. Initially patient can be with or without pain. The cellulitis and fracture can look alike. The condition needs examination by the doctor.

As the clot reaches the lung, then chest pain, cough with blood, shortness of breath, low blood pressure and passing out or collapse happens. The diagnosis is made with blood tests D dimer, clotting factors assay, hypoxemia, and arterial blood gas(ABG). Chest X-ray of the lungs may be normal.

DUPLEX SCAN of leg can be positive for DVT. The duplex is ultra sound test which shows blood flow and structure of vein. Ventilation perfusion(VQ) scan shows mismatch. Magnetic resonance imaging(MRI) is done in pregnant woman to avoid radiation exposure.

Pulmonary Angiogram is very sensitive to diagnose PE. TREATMENT is: THROMBOLYSIS by clot buster VENA CAVA FILTER, if the clot buster is contraindicated. SURGICAL EMBOLECTOMY is done with either thrombolysis failed or contraindicated.

**NOTE:** If there is acute onset of one leg swelling with tenderness, go to emergency room and get **DUPLEX OF LEG**. Use of blood thinner if indicated. Weight reduction. Keep on moving, no constant sitting . Take break after one hour for 5 minutes. learn to do exercise in the chair.

# PNEUMONIA:

The chest pain of pneumonia can be sometimes similar to heart attack in severity and location. it can be sharp like stabbing. It can cause heart attack. The patient can have fever, productive cough with yellow, green or rusty sputum, nausea, vomiting, shortness of breath and weakness.

May have headaches & confusion. Surprisingly the elderly people do not show symptoms because of their weak immune system. They are generally weak and confused.

It is the bacterial, viral or fungal infection of lung. It is contagious and spreads by person to person.

The diagnosis is made by History and physical examination.
CHEST X-ray shows the infiltrate/ pneumonia.
The blood tests are: Complete blood count (CBC). Comprehensive metabolic panel (CMP). 2 sets of blood cultures. Procalcitonin level. CRP and Sed Rate. PT/INR. Blood lactate level for infection.

The treatment of Pneumonia is:
- Appropriate broad spectrum antibiotic initially and later culture sensitive antibiotic
- Symptomatic. For fever Tylenol, and cough Robitussin.
- Oral fluid or IV hydration.

# PNEUMOTHORAX

It is known as collapsed lung. The chest pain is acute sudden, and sharp with shortness of breath. The air leaks from the lungs and goes into the space outside the body. It increases the pressure in the pleural space, and decreases the lung volume. The Normal pressure is negative.

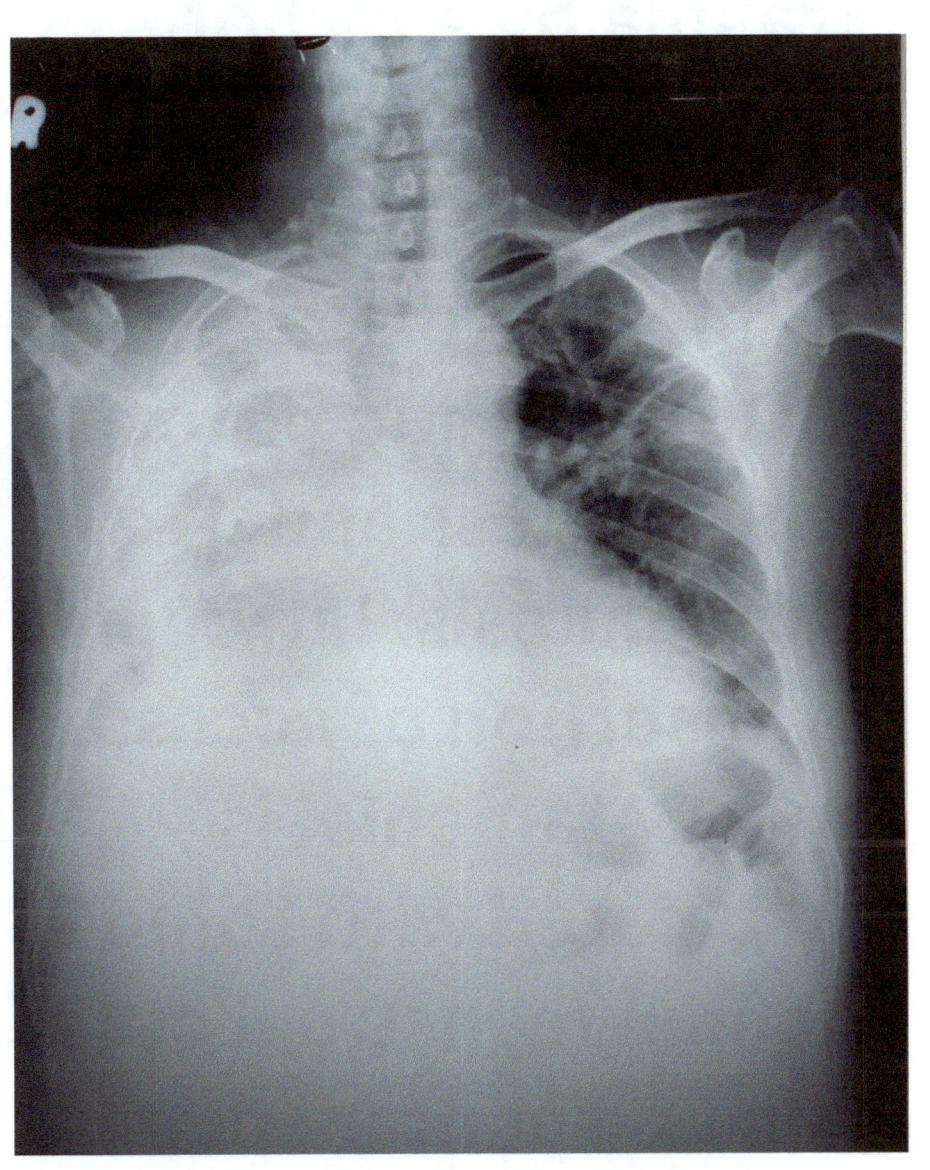

**PNEUMOTHORAX**

Causes:
Trauma by gunshot, stab, or car accident. Chronic obstructive pulmonary disease (COPD), Cystic fibrosis, lung abscess and Tuberculosis. Iatrogenic by insertion of access line. Catamenial is associated with some women menstrual cycle. Can be spontaneous with no cause

**TREATMENT:**
In the symptomatic patient immediate needle insertion, or pigtail catheter, or chest tube placement.

IV pain medications are administered.

It can be recurrent.
**IT CAN BE A REAL EMERGENCY, SO RUSH TO THE HOSPITAL.**

# PEPTIC ULCER DISEASE:

The pain of stomach ulcer is burning or dull and looks like heart attack. Ulcer is actually open sore in the stomach wall.
Pain is located in the area below breast bone or in the back, and can be aggravated by food, Ibuprofen, Naprosyn, and Aspirin etc.

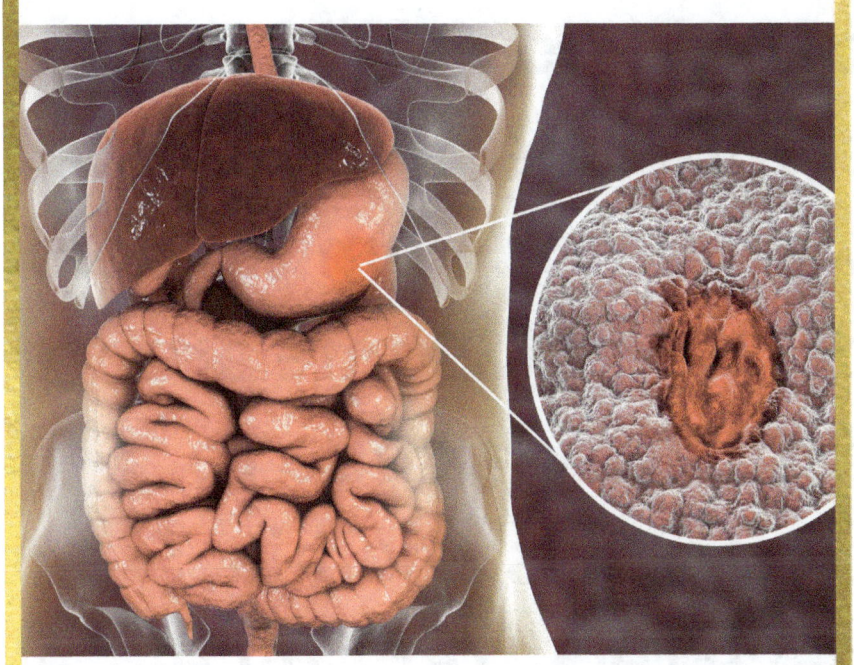

# PEPTIC ULCER DISEASE

It can be associated with belching, nausea, vomiting, and abdominal discomfort. Some people do not have any symptoms. Some come with blood vomiting or dark stool. Some are tired & weak due to blood loss anemia. Some have recurrent ulcer, and patient knows the history.

The causes of Peptic Ulcer disease are Infection by H. pylori, or drugs like Naprosyn, Advil, or any other NSAIDs, high acid secreting tumors like Hypergastrinemia or ZES, Zollinger-Ellison syndrome.

In the hospital, patients on ventilators for more than 48 hours develope ulcer, as the body is under the stress.
Alcohol and smoking can cause it.

The diagnosis of PUD
Urea breath testing, serology for for H. pylori
UGI ( UPPER GASTROINTESTIN AL) series.
EGD or upper endoscopy
Modified barium swallow study
pH monitoring is the gold standard.

Treatment:
- H. pylori treatment with triple medical regimen.
- Discontinue offending drugs
- Surgery vagotomy for refractory ulcer, that is done less now a days.

The complications are serious bleeding, perforation or stricture.
Treatment:

Life style modifications should be, to avoid alcohol, smoking, fatty food, sugary drinks.

Discontinue NSAID pain killer medications and other offending drugs.

Take Vit.c, probiotic and do weight reduction.

# ACID REFUX:

The stomach produces 3-4 liters of ydrochloric acid daily.

The acidity is measured in pH, on scale of 1 to 13 (1 being extremely acid, 7 being neutral and 13 being alkaline). The pH of stomach is 3, which is very acidic. The acid is neutralized by bicarbonate and mucous membrane.

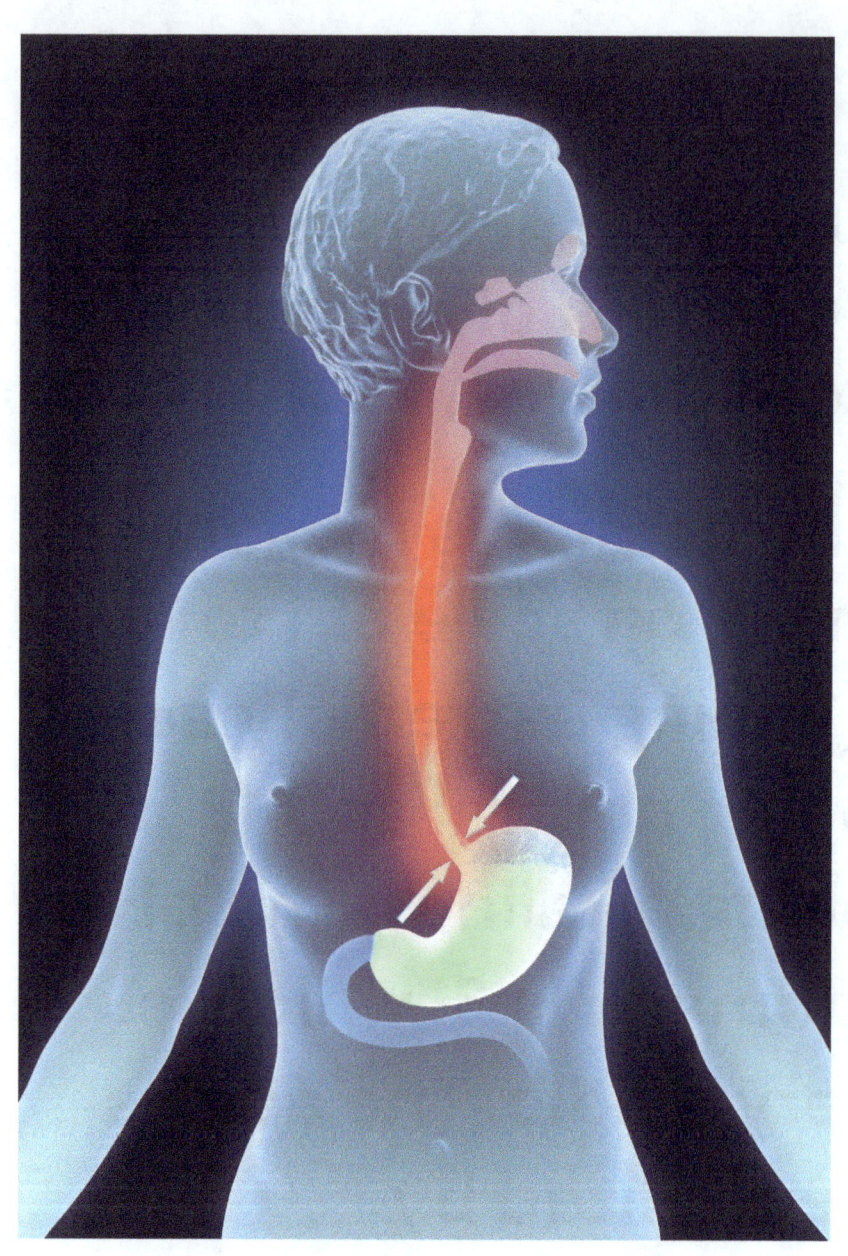

**ACID REFLUX DISEASE
GERD**

The acid function is to start predigestion process, absorbs calcium, magnesium, iron and B12, and kills bacteria. Acid is contained in the stomach and causes no harm because of natural bicarbonate and mucous membrane protection.

The predigested food goes to small intestine.

Acid reflux is also known as GERD or the gastro esophageal reflux disease. The pain of acid reflux is like angina or heart attack. It is burning and squeezing in chest .It may be associated with cough and sore throat. The sign and symptoms include mild to moderate chest pain specially after large meal with some type of regurgitation.

Causes of acid reflux.
Obesity
Hiatal hernia
Fatty food
Alcohol
Smoking
Chocolate
Prescribed medications are: iron, opioids, antibiotics etc.

**TREATMENT:** Abstain from smoking, drinking, caffeine, and prescribed offending drugs. Life style modifications should include weight reduction and fatty food avoidance.

Small portion protein meals. Take 3-4 hours, after dinner, to go to bed. No mid night snack. Head elevation at 45 degrees in bed. Use Pepcid(Famotidine) or Protonix (Pantoprazole)

Upper endoscopy to see other causes.

## GALL STONE:

The pain of gall stone is severe, sharp in right upper abdomen, and mimics the heart attack. The pain can be squeezing or stabbing. It can last from minutes to hours. It can radiate to the shoulder.

It can be associated with nausea, vomiting, light color stool, jaundice, or fever.

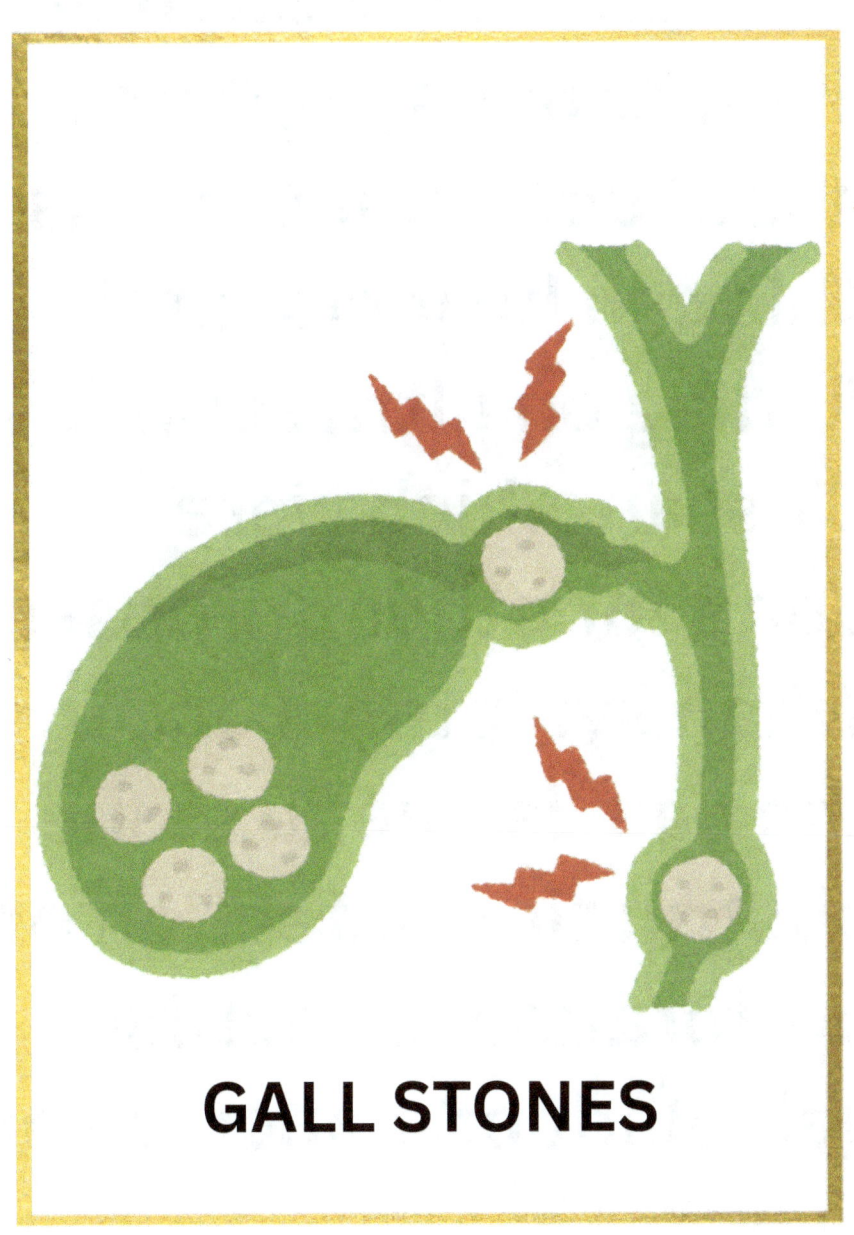

**GALL STONES**

Some people can have gall stone all their life without symptoms. It is *silent cholelithiasis*. This can be incidental finding on ultra sound, CT scan which were done for other purposes. When symptoms occur, the pain is due to stone obstruction, infection or perforation, effecting gall bladder, pancreas or liver.

The diagnostic tests are :
- Liver function and CBC blood tests
- Ultra sound of gall bladder.
- X-RAY of abdomen
- HIDA scan.
- MRI.
- ERCP.

The complications of gall stone are: obstruction with sepsis jaundice, pancreatitis cholecystitis, cholangitis
Small chance of cancer with gall stone.
Bowel obstruction can be serious complication.

Treatment:
- Mostly laparoscopic surgery, if patient is symptomatic.
- If patient is stable, asymptomatic and does not want elective surgery then medication Actigal (ursodiol) can be used for long time, usually at least 2 years.

**INSTRUCTIONS:**

Eat fruits, vegetables, whole wheat, low fat dairy products. Avoid fatty fast food, soda and sugary drinks. Small meals 4-5 times a day. Use of lemon, fish and olive oil. This diet prevents pain recurrence. Try weight loss.

# COSTOCHONDRITIS

It is the inflammation of cartilage which joins rib with breast bone. It is also known as anterior chest wall syndrome. Person feels pain after strenuous exercise, and worsens with breathing. The exact cause is not known.

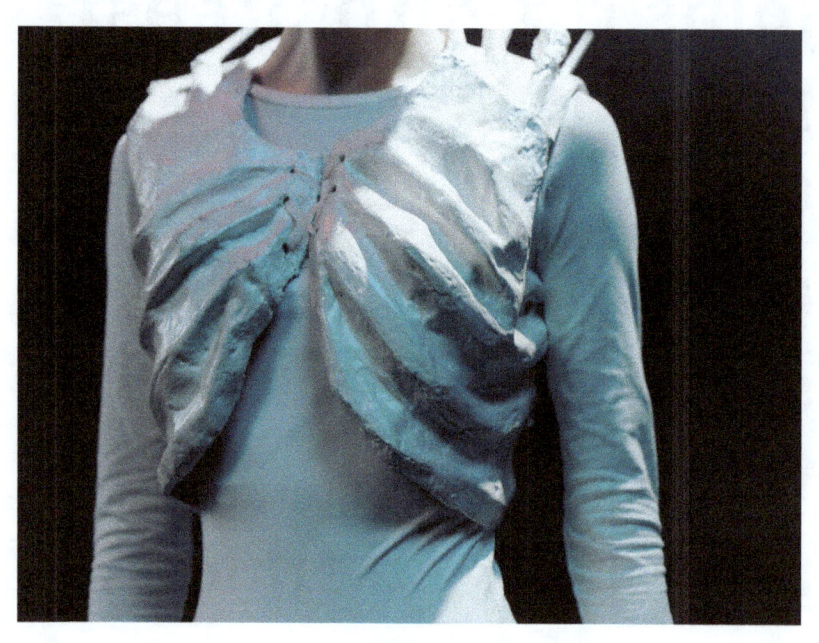

# COSTOCHNDRITIS

The pain is acute, severe, sharp, left side at once and can radiat to shoulder or left arm like heart attack. It is aggravated by the deep breathing, and chest pressure after strenuous exercise . Can be felt by putting single finger on joint and will reproduce the tenderness.

No specific diagnostic tests for costochondritis because the tests are first done for other serious chest pain diseases and applied for costochondritis, as it is the diagnosis of exclusion. Those tests are basic CBC, CMP, chest X-RAY, ECG, Ultra sound etc.

**TREATMENT:**

Is rest mostly and pain management with NSAIDS, CAPSAICIN, LIDOCAINE PATCH and DICLOFENAC GEL. Vitamin D is given if there is deficiency. Treat underlying disease.

It gets better in short term mostly, but can linger on for a while.

## ANXIETY:

Anxiety is a constant worry, apprehension, fear, exaggerated thinking of about every day situations and events. Person is edgy with blank mind. This state is going on for about 3-6 months. The thinking and behavior of person are effected. It is due to imbalance of neurotransmitters.

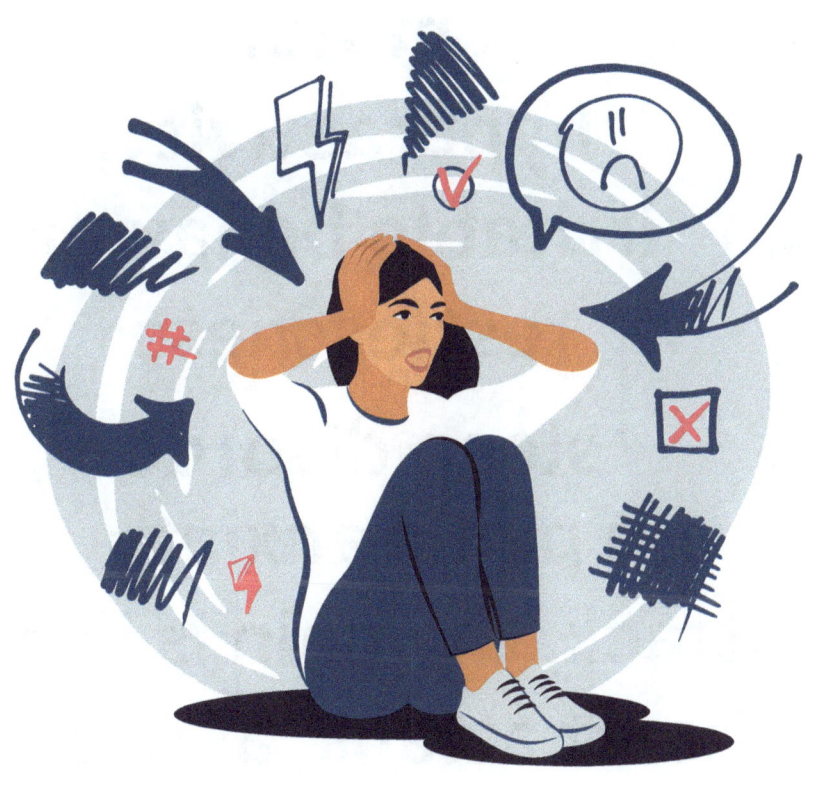

# ANXIETY

97

The person has
- cognitive vigilance
- forgetfulness
- motor hyperactivity,
- irritable behavior
- restlessness
- sleep disorder

In panic anxiety attack, the pain is like heart attack, at mid sternum but does radiates to arm.

Panic attack is short periodic intense anxiety, fear of apprehension with racing heart, perspiration weakness, fainting, shaking, tingling sensation in hand or feet, depersonalization or dying feeling. Actually there is no real danger

Beside that, anxiety has spectrum of Obsessive compulsive disorder(OCD), with uncontrollable recurring thoughts and behavior. Post traumatic stress disorder(PTSD), with flash back of traumatic events. The diagnostic and statistical manual of mental disorders (DSM) has classified them as separate entities now.

## TREATMENT

- Avoid caffeine, alcohol and recreational drugs.
- FOCUS on regular diet, deep breathing, yoga, exercise and good sleep.
- COGNITIVE BEHAVIOR THERAPY.
- Medications mostly Benzodiazepines & SSRI. Psych. F/U.
-